How To Avoid a Bear Attack

Mastering The Art of Avoidance and Survival: Know, Prevent, Survive, And What to Do If You Encounter a Bear, Playing Dead - When and How, And Safety Equipment and Tools

Kobo Press

Disclaimer:

Please note that the information contained in this book is intended solely for educational purposes. The information contained in this book was obtained from a wide variety of different sources.

By continuing to read this document, the reader acknowledges and agrees that the author is in no way responsible for any losses, whether indirect or direct, that may be incurred as a direct or indirect result of the information presented in this book, including but not limited to omissions and errors.

Contents

Introduction 4

Different Bear Species....................................6

Bears Habitat and Behavior 10

Preventing Bear Attacks 13

Understanding Bear Psychology 21

What To Do If You Encounter a Bear 29

Surviving A Bear Attack..............................37

Tools And Safety Equipment 44

First Aid for Bear Encounters 49

Introduction

In the heart of the wilderness, where the ancient trees stand as silent sentinels and the rivers sing their timeless songs, there exists a primal dance between man and beast. Among the towering pines and rugged peaks, one creature commands both respect and fear: the bear.

In these pages, embark on a journey of discovery and empowerment, equipping you with the knowledge and skills to outwit, evade, and, if necessary, survive encounters with one of nature's most formidable predators.

Bears, with their majestic presence and fierce demeanor, evoke a sense of awe and reverence. Yet, beneath their charismatic exterior lies a complex world of instincts, behaviors, and territorial boundaries.

Through meticulous research and expert insight, unravel the mysteries of bear psychology, offering a window into the minds of these enigmatic creatures.

But knowledge alone is not enough. In "How to avoid a bear attack", this guide goes beyond theory to provide practical strategies and creative solutions for avoiding bear encounters altogether. From proper food storage techniques to choosing safe campsites, youre armed with the tools needed to navigate the wilderness with confidence and foresight.

The possibility of a bear encounter looms ever-present, but in these moments of peril, this guide serves as your lifeline, offering step-by-step guidance on how to react with calmness, clarity and prepare you for the unexpected, to face the unknown with courage and resilience.

But " How to avoid a bear attack " is more than just a survival manual; It is the journey into the heart of bear country, unlock the secrets of survival, and forge a deeper bond with the wild places that call to our souls.

With this guide, the adventure begins now.

Different Bear Species

It is essential to comprehend the many bear species to appreciate their roles in the ecosystem and to be able to safely navigate their habitats. Bear safety should be approached with consideration for the distinct habits, diets, and habitats of each species.

An overview of the eight bear species you might come across or hear about is given in this chapter.

Black bear in America (Ursus americanus)

The most prevalent and extensively dispersed bear species in North America is the American black bear. Although they might be brown or blonde, they are usually black.

Habitat: Found in hilly areas, wetlands, and woodlands from Alaska to Mexico in North America.

Food: An omnivore's diet consists of fish, plants, fruits, insects, and small mammals. They have a reputation for stealing food from campers and human waste.

Behavior: Usually timid and non-aggressive around people, but if they become accustomed to eating humans, they may become assertive. They are skilled ascensionists.

Ursus arctos, or brown bear

Brown bears range in color from light brown to dark brown and are big, strong animals. Among the subspecies are the well-known Kodiak bear (Ursus arctos Middendorf) and Grizzly bear (Ursus arctos horribilis).

Their habitat is varied, ranging from the tundra regions to the woods and mountains of North America and Eurasia.

Diet: Omnivorous, consuming berries, vegetables, animals, fish (particularly salmon), and fish. In coastal areas, grizzlies may have a high fish diet.

Behavior: Mostly solitary, except mating season and times when moms are with their young. They can be highly aggressive, especially when they're scared or trying to defend their cubs. renowned for having a hump on their shoulders and a strong physique.

Bear (Ursus maritimus) polar

The largest bear species, polar bears are distinguished by their white fur, which helps them blend in with their Arctic surroundings.

Habitat: In the Arctic, which includes the coasts of Canada, Alaska, Russia, Greenland, and Norway, they are mainly found on sea ice.

Eats mostly carnivorous foods, such as seals. Sea ice is necessary for them to reach their prey.

Behavior: Excellent swimmers and very acclimated to chilly settings. all but alone, except mothers and cubs. Because of their size and raptors' instincts, they may pose a threat to people.

Black Bear (Ursus thibetanus) in Asia

Because of the white marking in the shape of a crescent on its breast, it is often referred to as the moon bear. Their black fur is shaggy.

Found in woods and hilly regions of Asia, such as Southeast Asia, Japan, and the Himalayas.

Omnivorous: Consumes fruits, nuts, insects, and small animals as part of its diet.

Behavior: They are adept climbers and are often nocturnal and arboreal. When threatened or when their cubs are in danger, they may become aggressive.

Tremarctos ornatus, the Andean Bear

The only bear species that is native to South America is the Andean bear, also known as the spectacled bear. They feature characteristic, glasses-like patterns surrounding their eyes.

Habitat: Dwell in the high Andes highlands and cloud forests of Bolivia, Ecuador, Peru, Colombia, and Venezuela.

Food: Omnivorous; mainly consists of fruits and bromeliads, with the occasional small animal.

Behavior: They spend most of their time in trees and are solitary and evasive in general. less hostile than other bears towards people.

Ailuropoda melanoleuca, or panda bear

Description: One of the most known and adored bear species is pandas, which are distinguished by their unique black-and-white coloring.

Habitat: Native to bamboo woods in central China.

Diet: Mostly bamboo, though they also sometimes consume carrion and small animals.

Behavior: They spend most of their time eating bamboo and are solitary and calm. Because of their low reproduction rates and disappearing habitat, they are deemed fragile.

The Melursus ursinus, or sloth bear

Sloth bears are characterized by their long, shaggy fur and a noticeable white or yellowish mark on their breast. They eat differently—by sucking insects with their lips.

The Indian subcontinent is home to a variety of habitats, including grasslands and forests.

Food: Mostly insectivorous, consuming fruits and honey in addition to termites and ants.

Behavior: They are nocturnal and renowned for their fierce self-defense when cornered. They walk slowly and deliberately, and they are great climbers.

Helarctos malayanus, the Sun Bear

The smallest kind of bear, distinguished by a white or orange patch on its breast and short black fur. They can extract insects and honey with their lengthy tongues.

Habitat: Found in Southeast Asian tropical forests, encompassing Borneo, Sumatra, and the Malay Peninsula.

Omnivorous: Consumes fruits, insects, tiny vertebrates, and honey among other foods.

Behavior: Mostly solitary and arboreal. renowned for their natural shyness and tree-climbing dexterity.

Comprehending the distinctions between various bear species is essential for both conservation and safety purposes. Understanding these amazing animals' habitats, food, and behaviors enables us to coexist with them while reducing hazards and advancing their preservation.

Bears Habitat and Behavior

To prevent bear encounters and to recognize the importance of bears in the environment, it is essential to comprehend the habitats and habits of the various bear species.

Habitats for Common Bears

Woods:

Forested regions are ideal for many bear species, such as the Asian Black Bear, Brown Bear, and American Black Bear. In addition to offering many food items including fruits, nuts, and small animals, these environments also offer cover for dens and protection.

Mountains:

Mountainous areas are home to brown bears, particularly grizzlies, who may access a variety of food sources and have ideal denning terrain. Mountainous regions of the Andes are also home to Andean Bears.

Coastal and Tundra Regions:

Because of their adaptation to the Arctic tundra and coastal areas, polar bears hunt seals on sea ice. In areas like Alaska, where salmon runs offer essential food, brown bears also depend heavily on coastal environments.

Savannas and Grasslands:

In the Indian subcontinent's grasslands and savannas, where they can dig for insects and fruits, sloth bears are frequently encountered.

Tropical Woods:

Tropical forests are home to Sun Bears and Andean Bears, who can eat a wide range of fruits and insects there. There is plenty of protection and food in these lush forests.

Forests of bamboo:

Because bamboo is such an abundant food supply in these bamboo forests in central China, giant pandas have evolved specific adaptations for surviving there.

Bear Habits and Seasonal Trends

Winter hibernation:

Throughout the winter, many bear species, including the American Black Bear and Brown Bear, hibernate. Bears go into a state of reduced metabolic activity at this time to save energy if food becomes scarce.

Feeding Patterns:

Bears are opportunistic feeders, and their diets change according to the season and species. For example, American Black Bears browse for berries and nuts in late summer and fall, while Brown Bears may rely mostly on salmon during the spawning season.

The concept of territoriality

Bears may be territorial and usually have huge home ranges. While female bears with cubs may be more protective of their region, male bears frequently have broader territories that overlap with multiple females.

Cubs and Reproduction:

Bears often mate in late spring or early summer, though this varies depending on the species. Usually, one to four cubs are born to female bears during hibernation or in the den throughout the winter. Bear mothers fiercely defend their offspring, and they may become especially hostile if they feel that their cubs are in danger.

Denning

Bears choose den locations that offer safety and weather protection. Dens can be found underground, in hollow trees, or caverns. Early on in their lives, cub survival depends heavily on the den site they choose.

Identifying Bear Indications: Footprints, Scat, and Markings

Tracks:

Bear footprints are unique in that they have five toes and obvious claws. While brown bears have longer, straighter claws for digging, American black bears have more curled claws that are more adapted for climbing.

Scattered

Bear scat differs according to nutrition. It may have plant debris, hair, bones, or berry fragments. Determining the presence and activity level of bears in the region might be aided by identifying scat.

Notations:

Bears use a variety of marking techniques to identify their territory, including clawing, rubbing, and scent marking. Bear activity and presence in a region can be inferred from these markings.

Preventing Bear Attacks

Preventing confrontations with bears is the greatest method to assure safety when in bear territory. Bears tend to stay away from people, but some behaviors can draw them near or put you at risk.

This chapter goes over the fundamentals of hiking and camping, including how to store food properly and manage waste, use bear-resistant containers, travel in groups, make noise, and select safe campsites.

By adhering to these recommendations, bear encounter risks can be reduced and human and bear safety can be enhanced.

The Greatest Techniques for Camping and Hiking

Go in Groups

Larger groups are less likely to be approached by bears. Plan your outdoor adventures so that you can trek or camp with a minimum of four people. Bears find larger groups more threatening, which lowers the likelihood of a bear encounter. Furthermore, organizations can support one another in an emergency.

Create Sound

When trekking, it's important to make noise to keep bears from startling you. Like many other wild creatures, bears prefer to stay away from people and will frequently retreat if they hear you approaching.

Sing, clap your hands, talk loudly, or use bear bells when vision is poor or in densely vegetated areas. You should speak up more in windy areas near boisterous streams so that bears can hear you from a distance.

Follow Recognized Trails

Because bears are less likely to use well-traveled trails than off-trail places, using them can lessen the chance of coming across them. You can see bears from a distance on established paths since they have less dense foliage and better visibility.

Keep an Eye Out

Keep an eye on your surroundings at all times. Keep an eye out for bear evidence on trees, such as tracks, scat, and claw marks. It's advisable to go in the opposite direction or turn around if you see new signage. Always have binoculars on hand to look ahead for bear activity, particularly in meadows and open spaces.

Keep Bear Spray on Hand

A vital piece of equipment for bear country protection is bear spray. Make sure it is in a place where it is easy to get to, such as a holster on your belt or backpack strap. Practice releasing the safety clip and become proficient with its use. A violent bear can be deterred by bear spray, giving you time to get away and safe.

Don't go hiking at dusk or dawn.

When they are out foraging for food, bears are most active around dawn and dusk. When bear activity is reduced during the day, try to schedule your hikes around that time.

If you have to hike early in the morning or late at night, pay closer attention, be noisier, and remain aware of your surroundings.

Take Care When Using Pets

Bears can be agitated or attracted to pets, particularly dogs. If you bring a pet, make sure it is always under control and on a leash. Lost pets can help a bear find their way back to you. It may be advisable to leave pets at home in certain bear environments.

Steer clear of strong scents

Because of their keen sense of smell, bears are drawn to powerful scents. Steer clear of perfumes, deodorants, and lotions with scents. Strong-smelling non-food objects can also attract a bear's attention.

Learn for Yourself

Learn about the particular bear species you might come into before heading out into bear country.

Understanding the unique behaviors of various species will enable you to respond to them effectively when you come into contact with them.

Appropriate Food Preservation and Waste Handling

Bear-Proof Containers

Bear-resistant containers should be used to store all food, hygiene, and fragrant things. Bears are drawn to food from great distances due to their keen sense of smell. Bears are not supposed to be able to access the contents of these containers.

Hang Food

If bear-resistant storage isn't an option, hang your food with a rope at least ten feet above the ground and four feet away from any tree trunks. Bears are unable to climb or stand on their hind legs to get to it because of this. Make sure the food is tightly sealed in odor-proof bags to help minimize the stink.

Tidy campsites

Immediately wipe up any spills or food remnants to keep the campsite tidy. Steer clear of eating or cooking close to where you sleep. Cooking supplies and utensils should be hung with your food or kept in bear-proof containers.

Get Rid of Waste Correctly

Remove any rubbish and, if possible, dispose of it in bear-proof containers. Never burn or bury food scraps since bears may still be drawn to the smell. Wash dishes and use biodegradable soap away from where you sleep.

Applying Containers Resistant to Bears

Container Types

There are several different types of bear-resistant containers, such as soft-sided bags with strengthened closures and hard-sided canisters.

Select a container that meets both your demands and the rules in your area. Certain kinds of containers could be needed in certain places.

Appropriate Utilization

Make sure to store containers out of the way of sleeping areas and to properly close them. To stop bears from taking the container, place it on the ground or fasten it to something sturdy. For best results, use as directed by the manufacturer; incorrect use can lessen their effectiveness.

Accessible

For information about bear-resistant container availability and regulations, get in touch with your local land management organization. Certain parks and wilderness areas have leasing policies available, or their use is subject to rules. Make sure you have the right container for your vacation by planning beforehand.

Arrangement of Containers

Bears who are interested in your bear-resistant containers may tip them over or roll them away, so place them on level, firm ground. To prevent bears from moving the containers, try to anchor them with logs or rocks.

Community Standards

When it comes to bear-resistant containers, abide by local community norms and restrictions in places where camping is popular. Bear-resistant storage lockers may be available at campsites in certain parks and wilderness regions, subject to particular restrictions.

Learn about the particular kind of bear-resistant container you want to use before your journey. To open and close it fast and effectively in the field, practice doing so.

Making Noise and Traveling in Groups

Devices that Produce Noise

To let bears know you're about, use bear bells, air horns, or other noise-making equipment. These can be especially helpful in areas with a lot of greenery or close to waterways when vision is poor. Bear bells can make a continuous sound, but you need also talk loudly or clap frequently to make sure bears can hear you.

Group Interactions

Remain together as a group when traveling; especially in bear-prone areas, and avoid splitting off. Hiking in a tight formation is recommended, with the most experienced member leading and another experienced member trailing behind. This arrangement facilitates the management of interactions and emergencies by preserving group cohesion and noise levels.

Hold your children close.

Keep kids close and visible at all times when hiking with them. Youngsters might not understand the warning signs of a bear or how to respond safely. Inform them about bear safety and what to do in case of a bear encounter.

Remain Vigilant

Making noise is vital, but so is being aware of your surroundings and always attentive. Look forward and examine the area for any indications of bear activity, including noises, movement, or recently fallen sap.

Get Ready to Apply Bear Spray

Learn how to get and use your bear spray fast. Practice aiming and removing the safety clip. Bear spray should only be used as a last resort when a bear is charging or acting violently because it works best at a distance of 20 to 30 feet.

Selecting Secure Campsites

Steer clear of bear habitats

Pick campsites far from places where bears can find plenty of food, like berry bushes, streams where salmon are spawning, or places where carcasses have been found. As they look for food, bears are more likely to be spotted in these regions.

Secure Distances

At least 100 yards should separate your camp from the area where you prepare and store food. This distance reduces the possibility that the smell of food will draw a bear to your sleeping quarters. Make sure that your sleeping place is downwind from your cooking area and food storage area.

Seeing

Pick parking areas with good visibility. Steer clear of heavy plants and undergrowth where bears might be resting or feeding. You can identify bears at a distance and take proper action when you are in open places with unobstructed lines of sight.

Steer clear of game trails

Avoid camping close to bear routes or game pathways. These trails are frequently used by bears and camping close by increases the chance of a bear encounter. Select a location away from the main wildlife routes and keep an eye out for bear activity indicators.

Safe Campsite Boundaries

If you have access to electrified bear fences or tripwires with noise makers, set up a perimeter of bear deterrents around your campground. By warning you of a bear's presence or preventing it from accessing the camp, these can give an extra degree of security.

Think About Wind Direction

Consider the direction of the wind while arranging your campsite. To prevent food smells from leaking into your tent, place your cooking station downwind from where you sleep.

Elevation of Camp

Camp higher up if at all possible. Bears frequently follow low-lying terrain and river valleys, especially when they are on the lookout for food. Elevations above sea level may lessen the chance of coming across a bear.

Visibility and Lighting

Maintain good nighttime lighting at your campground by using lanterns and headlights. Bright lights can help you spot bears and dissuade them from approaching. Always have a flashlight on hand.

Barrier Techniques

If bear activity is high where you camp, you might want to use portable electric fences. Bears are successfully kept away from your tent and areas where you store food thanks to the powerful deterrent provided by these fences.

Plans for Emergencies

Establish an emergency plan. Find out where the closest places are to get aid or medical support. Make sure everyone in your group is aware of the emergency procedures in the event of a bear encounter, and always carry a map and compass.

It takes a proactive strategy that combines awareness, planning, and regular activities to prevent bear encounters. You may drastically lower your chances of coming across a bear by following the recommended hiking and camping procedures.

You must manage your waste and store food properly if you want bears to stay away from your campsite. Bears cannot obtain human food if bear-resistant containers are used successfully and regularly, which can save both human and bear lives.

Creating noise and going in groups are two easy but efficient ways to draw a bear's attention and lessen the chance of an encounter. To further assure your safety, pick well-lit, bear-resistant campsites that are away from bear habitats and transit routes. You should also practice proper camp hygiene.

Never forget that limiting bear interactions is about protecting bears' natural behaviors and reducing their acclimatization to humans, in addition to your safety. Bears that have gotten habituated may exhibit increased aggression and may need to be put down for the protection of people.

Respect these amazing critters' natural habitat while you appreciate the wilderness. You have the power to ensure that bears and humans live in harmony and that both species can prosper in their natural habitats by taking meaningful action.

To help with the conservation and safety of both wildlife and human visitors, always be aware, ready, and watchful.

Understanding Bear Psychology

It is essential to comprehend bear psychology to prevent bear interactions and deal with them appropriately when they do occur. Understanding bear behavior will help you make more accurate predictions about how they will respond in certain scenarios.

Bear territoriality and denning practices, feeding patterns (particularly about interactions with human food), and special safety measures required while interacting with mother bears and their offspring are all covered in this chapter.

Boundaries and Bear Dens

1. Recognizing territoriality

Bears are primarily solitary creatures with well-delineated areas, though the extent and intersection of these domains can differ greatly according to the species, gender, and habitat.

Home Range: The territory that a bear frequents to locate food, mate, and raise its young is known as its home range. The home ranges of male bears are usually bigger than those of female bears, and they frequently overlap multiple female' ranges. A male brown bear, for instance, might have a territory that spans hundreds of square kilometers.

Bears mark their territory by scent marking, vocalizing, and scratching trees. These techniques help the bears establish and express their presence. To leave a scent trail, they rub their bodies against trees, scratch, and occasionally urinate.

Intra-Species Communication: Bears can prevent direct conflicts with other bears by using these markers. Unless it's mating season or a quarrel over a rich food supply, a bear will typically choose to move away from another when it detects its scent or markings to avoid conflict.

2. Dens of Bears

Bear dens are essential for survival because they offer a secure location for cub rearing and protection during hibernation.

Bears choose their den locations depending on factors such as weather protection, insulation, and safety. Dens are located in excavated earth and snow dens, hollow trees, beneath logs, and caverns.

Hibernation: A bear's metabolism drastically slows down during hibernation, which can last anywhere from a few months to more than half the year, depending on the temperature. They don't eat, drink, urinate, or defecate during this time, although they are capable of waking up if they feel uneasy and may even momentarily leave the den.

Denning Behavior: In the spring, pregnant females usually emerge from their dens later with their young, having entered their dens earlier than males and non-pregnant females. They are extremely protective and vulnerable at this time.

3. Territory and Seasonal Movements

It is possible to anticipate where bears will be at different times of the year by having an understanding of the seasonal movements and changes in bear territory.

Spring: Bears are frequently hungry and on the lookout for food when they come out of hibernation. To locate the finest food supplies, such as fresh foliage or the remains of animals that perished in the winter, they may venture far within their range.

Summer: Bears' spheres of influence may slightly change as the summer goes on because they follow the availability of fruits, insects, and other food sources. Males may go farther in pursuit of partners.

Fall: Bears enter a condition of hyperphagia to accumulate fat reserves in preparation for hibernation. They might go a long way to locate bountiful food supplies, such as salmon streams or berry patches.

Winter: Bears stay in their dens while hibernating. Although they are usually dormant, disruptions can rouse them and even force them to emerge from the den, which can be hazardous for both humans and bears.

4. The Effect of Humans on Bear Areas

Bear behavior and territory can be greatly impacted by human activity.

Bear habitats can be overrun by development, logging, and recreational activities, which puts bears and people nearby. Meetings are more likely as a result of this.

Corridors and Connectivity: Bears depend on the preservation of natural corridors and connectivity between their many habitats. This keeps them safe from human development as they travel between locations in quest of food and partners.

Conservation Efforts: The long-term viability of bear populations depends on conservation initiatives that safeguard bear habitats and reduce human impact. This entails establishing wildlife corridors, designating protected areas, and instructing people on how to coexist peacefully with bears.

Habits of Feeding and Human Food

1. Organic Food

As omnivores, bears' diets differ greatly according to their species, location, and time of year. You can steer clear of circumstances where your presence might be interpreted as a competitor for resources by being aware of their feeding habits.

Diverse Diet: Plants, fruits, nuts, insects, fish, and tiny to large mammals are among the many items that bear eat. For example, polar bears mostly hunt seals, but black bears may consume a diet high in berries and insects.

Seasonal Variations: Depending on what's available throughout the year, bears modify their diets. They may eat winter-killed animal corpses and new growth in the spring. In the summer, bears typically consume a diet high in fruits and insects; in the fall, however, hyperphagia—the overindulgence in food necessary to store fat for hibernation—occurs.

2. Human Nutrition and Its Effects

Bear behavior can be significantly and dangerously affected by feeding from humans.

3. The Function of Overeating

A bear's feeding habits and relationships with humans are shaped during the crucial stage of hyperphagia in their life cycle.

Enhanced Activity: Bears are more active and spend a large portion of their time foraging during hyperphagia. More interactions with people may result from this increased activity, particularly in regions where human activity and natural food sources coexist.

Food Sources: Bears will eat everything that is highest in calories. This frequently includes trash, pet food, bird feeders, and carelessly stored camping food in areas where people are present.

Mitigation Strategies: Communities and individuals could lock up their trash, take down their bird feeders, and keep food in bear-proof containers to lower the chance of encounters during hyperphagia. Campaigns for public education can aid in increasing awareness of the significance of these actions.

4. Climate Change's Effects

Bear encounters with people are increasing and their eating habits are changing due to climate change.

Food Availability Shift: The time and availability of natural food supplies can be impacted by climatic changes. For instance, plant growth and prey animal movement patterns might be affected by early springs and warmer winters.

Range Expansion: Some bear species are moving into new regions as a result of rising temperatures, which may result in interactions with human populations who aren't used to coexisting with bears.

Adaptive Strategies: Although bears are incredibly adaptive animals, their capacity to locate natural food sources may be outpaced by the swift changes in their surroundings, increasing their dependence on food supplied by humans. Communities need to adjust by encouraging conservation initiatives and putting bear-aware behaviors into effect.

Bears are drawn to campsites by the aroma of trash and food left by humans. Their association of people with food can make them more aggressive and fearless in their pursuit of it.

Food Conditioning: Bears that have access to trash or human food can become desensitized to people and overcome their innate fear of them. This conduct frequently results in risky interactions and, regrettably, the bear's euthanasia to ensure the safety of humans.

Preventive measures include hanging food at suitable heights and distances from camp, storing food in bear-resistant containers, and carefully cleaning cooking areas to keep bears from developing a food-conditioned state.

Mother Bears and Cubs: Additional Safety Measures

1. Mother bears' protective nature

Mother bears, sometimes known as sows, are fiercely devoted to their young. For your safety, it is essential to comprehend this maternal instinct.

Maternal Aggression: A mother bear takes seriously any danger that might befall her cubs. She will react violently if she feels threatened. Her primary goal in being aggressive is to defend her young.

Cub rearing: During the one to three years that they spend with their moms, cubs pick up vital survival skills. The sow's behavior is concentrated on raising, nurturing, and safeguarding her young during this time.

2. Seeing a Sow with the Cubs

It's important to take extra care while approaching a mother bear with cubs to prevent inciting a defensive reaction.

Avoidance: If you spot cubs, move slowly backward, assuming the mother is not far away. Avoid trying to get close to or engage with the cubs as this will most likely result in the mother being combative.

Non-Threatening Behavior: You must behave in a non-threatening manner if a mother bear spots you. Steer clear of direct eye contact, talk quietly, and slowly wave your arms to enlarge yourself as you step back.

Climbing Trees: When scared, black bear cubs frequently climb trees. If you notice cubs in a tree, quickly get out of the area since the mother will be nearby, keeping an eye on the babies.

3. Safety precautions in cubby houses

Taking extra care will assist in ensuring safety when hiking or camping in places where mother bears and cubs are known to reside.

Increased Vigilance: During berry patches or fish-rich streams, places where mother bears and cubs are likely to be seen, use extra caution.

Traveling in Groups: As with any bear encounter, this can help prevent violent behavior. To indicate their presence, groups should stay near to one another and generate noise.

Knowledge and Preparation: Learn about the unique ways that mother bears in the area you are visiting behave. Keep bear spray on you and be proficient with its application in case of an encounter.

4. Recognizing Cub Signs

Recognizing the telltale indicators of cub presence will help you steer clear of potentially hazardous situations.

Scat and smaller footprints: Scat and smaller tracks can be signs that cubs are about. Seek indications that a sow has recently traversed a region with her cubs.

Noises: Cubs, particularly when they're upset, may be very talkative. If there are high-pitched whimpers or squeals, it's a good idea to exercise extra caution.

Climbing Trees: Cubs frequently scale trees to get away from danger. It's advisable to flee the area right once if you spot cubs in trees because the mother will probably be close by and quite protective.

5. Variations in Species Behavior

There are differences in the ways that different bear species protect their cubs and mother them.

American Black Bear: Mother black bears are generally more accepting of people, but they will still protect their young if they feel threatened. When they evaluate the circumstances, they are more likely to send their pups up a tree.

Brown/Grizzly Bear: Mothers of grizzly bears are well-known for fiercely defending their young. They are more prone to attack or charge people who they believe pose a threat to their young.

Polar Bear: When their pups are in danger, polar bear moms can become quite combative and protective. Because of their isolated environments, encounters are rare but extremely deadly.

Asian Black Bear: Like their American counterparts, these bears will defend their cubs fiercely if they feel threatened, frequently taking to trees as a haven for the young.

Sloth Bear: Sloth bear moms are extremely protective of their young and have been known to use force to protect them. They are also known for carrying their pups on their backs.

Sun Bear: Not much is known about their defense mechanisms, but just like other bear species, moms of sun bears would use force to protect their young when needed.

Andean Bear: Although these bears are usually shy, moms will aggressively defend their young against any perceived threats.

6. Human Relationships and Education

Reducing hazardous interactions between mother bears and their pups requires community involvement and education.

Community events: To educate the public about bear behavior and safety, local wildlife agencies and conservation organizations frequently provide events.

Engaging in these initiatives can yield useful data and resources.

Notifying Local Wildlife Authorities of Bear Sightings: Notify the local wildlife authorities of any sightings of a mother bear and her cubs. This can alert nearby residents to possible hazards and aid in tracking bear movements.

Bear Safety exercises: Being familiar with bear safety exercises, such as applying bear spray and handling a bear encounter, will help you respond to a mother bear and her kids in a composed and efficient manner.

You can prevent unintentionally invading bear territory by being aware of the telltale signals of their activity and showing respect for their territories. To stop bears from developing a food-conditioned response and associating people with simple meals, proper food storage, and waste management are crucial.

Dealing with mother bears and their cubs requires extra caution because of the mother's protective nature, which makes these interactions very risky. Reducing hazards and fostering cohabitation requires that you and others educate yourselves on bear behavior and safety precautions.

We can guarantee safer outdoor activities and support the conservation and well-being of these amazing animals by respecting bears and their natural behaviors. When in bear country, always stay alert, organized, and knowledgeable. Also, keep in mind that human actions can have a big impact on preserving a peaceful coexistence with the wildlife that shares our earth.

What To Do If You Encounter a Bear

Although seeing a bear in the outdoors can be frightening, the likelihood of getting hurt can be greatly decreased by being aware of the bear's behavior and knowing how to respond.

This chapter explores how to recognize various bear behavior patterns, what to do right away if you come across a bear, how to use bear spray effectively, and how to read body language.

Recognizing a Bear's Behavior: Inquisitive, Protective, or Predatory

Bears display a variety of behaviors according to the circumstances and their motivations. Being aware of these actions will enable you to react correctly.

1. Inquisitive Conduct

Usually investigating their surroundings, curious bears may approach people more out of curiosity than out of hostility.

Curiosity cues: A curious bear will stand erect and frequently stand on its hind legs to have a closer look or take a smell. It might move softly toward you, its ears pricked, its body at ease.

Appropriate Reaction: Communicate calmly and make yourself appear larger by waving your arms. Facing the bear, carefully back away and allow it plenty of room to escape.

2. Retaliatory Actions

When a bear feels threatened, it will defend itself, its cubs, or its food by acting violently.

Bears that exhibit defensive behavior may snort, clack their teeth, or huff. They could swat the ground, put their ears back, and droop their head. In a bluff show, a protective bear could also attack without really making contact.

Proper Reaction: Keep your cool and refrain from making abrupt gestures. Talk in a soothing, calm tone, and take a steady step back. Avoid running since this may lead to a pursuit reaction. Bear charges are sometimes bluff charges, so if the bear does, hold your ground.

3. Predatory Actions

Bear predators are uncommon but deadly. Usually, sick or food-conditioned bears exhibit this behavior.

Indicators of Predatory Behavior: A predatory bear will display a more intent and stalking demeanor, with its body stiff, head down, and ears forward. It might follow you stealthily and persistently.

Appropriate Reaction: If you witness predatory conduct, attempt to enlarge yourself and utilize all of your resources to project a sense of threat. Prepare to defend yourself with bear spray or any other available weaponry if the bear moves closer.

Take Action Right Away

The way you react to a bear encounter can make all the difference in how it turns out. Here's a detailed instruction manual to follow:

1. Remain composed.

Making bad choices can result from panic. Breathe deeply to de-stress and evaluate the circumstances.

2. Determine the Bear's Actions

To decide what to do next, quickly assess whether the bear is predatory, defensive, or inquisitive.

3. Identify Yourself

Talk in a steady, composed tone. You can demonstrate that you are a human and not an animal by slowly waving your arms.

4. Return Gradually

Without turning your back on the animal, steadily retreat. Keep your eyes open but avoid giving off a hostile stare.

5. Get Ready to Apply Bear Spray

Remove the safety clip from your bear spray and get ready in case the bear gets closer. For optimum control, hold the canister with both hands.

6. Remain Firm

Take a stand if the bear charges. Claims are mostly bluffs. When the bear is within 20 to 30 feet of you, use your bear repellent.

7. Defend Yourself

If a bear makes contact, shield your neck and head with your arms and, if it's a grizzly, pretend to be dead. If it's a black bear, fight back, focusing on the muzzle and face of the animal.

How to Apply Bear Spray Correctly

One of the best ways to dissuade hostile bears is using bear spray. It must be used properly to be effective.

1. Selecting the Appropriate Bear Spray

Make sure the bear spray you have is bear-specific and approved by the EPA. Bears cannot be effectively protected against common pepper sprays meant for human self-defense.

2. Having Bear Spray on the Hand

Keep your bear spray in a holster that is easy to reach. Even under pressure, you should be able to draw it rapidly and without stuttering.

3. Applying Bear Spray

Take off the Safety Clip: Take off the safety clip as soon as you see a bear getting closer.

Aim Low: To make a mist that the bear must pass through, aim slightly downward.

Spray in Bursts: Pull the trigger in quick bursts of one to two seconds, modifying your aim as necessary.

Hold Your Ground: Keep spraying until the bear moves away or in a different direction.

4. Following the Use of Bear Spray

Remove yourself from the area right away. Bear spray is extremely irritating, and once the effects wear off, the afflicted region may attract the bear again.

Report: File a report with the local authorities, particularly if the bear was food-conditioned or exhibiting violent behavior.

How to Apply Bear Spray Correctly

In an aggressive bear encounter, bear spray is your best line of protection, but it's only useful when applied properly.

1. Correct Methodology

Position: For improved stability and accuracy, hold the canister with both hands.

Bear spray has an effective range of twenty to thirty feet. Don't deploy until the bear is within this range.

Aim Low: To guarantee that the spray creates a cloud that the bear must pass through, aim slightly downward.

Controlled Bursts: Pull the trigger in quick bursts of one to two seconds. This produces a denser cloud and conserves your spray.

Spray Constantly: If the bear keeps coming closer, keep spraying, focusing on its face.

2. Following the Meeting

After utilizing the spray, quickly remove yourself from the area. The bear may move away for a while, but as the effects wear off, it may come back.

Report the Incident: Let the regional wildlife authorities know that bear spray was used and that an interaction occurred. This makes tracking bear behavior and any trouble spots easier.

3. Bear Spray in Various Situations

Wind: Recognize the direction of the wind. If at all feasible, spray downwind to prevent spray from blowing back at you.

Cold Weather: In very cold temperatures, bear spray canisters may not function as intended. Carry the canister near to your body to maintain its warmth.

Multiple Bears: Prioritize spraying the closest or most hostile bear first in the rare instances when there are multiple bears.

Recognizing the Body Language of Bears

Understanding a bear's body language can help you react appropriately and provide important insights into the bear's intentions.

1. Position and Motion

Bears frequently rise upright on their hind legs to gain a better perspective or to sniff the surroundings. Usually, this is a sign of curiosity rather than hostility.

Ears: While relaxed ears imply a protective or combative stance, erect ears convey interest or attention.

Head Position: When combined with vocalizations, a lowered head is frequently indicative of hostility.

2. Voices

Huffing and Popping: As a warning, bears emit sounds like huffing, popping, or jaw-clicking. This is a bear on the defensive, trying to get you to back off.

Roaring and Growling: Intense vocalizations such as roaring and growling suggest increased hostility and the possibility of an assault.

3. Maintain Eye Contact

Direct Eye Contact: Making direct eye contact might be difficult. It is advisable to maintain visual contact with the bear rather than confronting it head-on.

Bears that look as though they are concentrating on food or other tasks and avoid making eye contact are less likely to feel frightened.

4. Particular Actions

Bluff Charging: Bears may charge at you, only to abruptly turn away. This is meant to intimidate you and establish authority. Keep your distance and have bear spray ready.

Bears that swat the ground or stomp indicate that they are agitated and trying to get your attention.

Nose Down and Circling: Stealthy bears may move in a stalking manner, gliding silently while circling and lowering their noses to evaluate potential prey like you. Make yourself look bigger in this situation, and be ready to protect yourself.

Comprehending the body language of bears, including their posture, vocalizations, and distinct actions, might yield important insights into their intents and facilitate proper responses.

You may lessen the possibility of a dangerous encounter and raise your chances of having a positive and safe bear-viewing experience by being well-informed and prepared.

It's critical to know how to respond if you encounter a bear. Here's a more thorough explanation of what you should do right away in light of the various bear behaviors we previously covered.

1. Meeting an Inquisitive Bear

Keep Your Cool: Try not to flinch or make quick movements that could frighten an inquisitive bear.

Talk strongly but Gently: Show the bear that you are a human by speaking strongly yet softly.

Slow Motion: To make yourself appear bigger, wave your arms slowly above your head.

Back Away: Gradually retreat from the bear while keeping eye contact. Don't back down or flee.

2. Coming Upon a Protective Bear

Remain Still: If the bear is acting defensively or seems upset, do not move and remain motionless.

Communicate: Keep speaking to the bear in a gentle, collected tone.

Evaluate the situation by keeping an eye on the bear's actions to determine whether it is growing calmer or more upset.

Slow Retreat: While facing the bear, gradually back away if it seems to be relaxing. Don't back down or flee.

Be Ready for Bluff Charges: Anticipate a bluff charge from the bear. Remain motionless, as sprinting may result in a pursuit reaction.

3. Coming Across a Predatory Bear

Be Assertive: React aggressively if the bear is acting in a predatory manner. Make an effort to appear as big and menacing as you can while shouting and waving your arms.

Use Objects: To make oneself appear larger, use whatever items you own, such as a jacket or backpack.

Bear Spray Ready: If the bear keeps getting closer, have your bear spray ready to go.

Fight Back: If the bear attacks, strike back forcefully, concentrating on the face and muzzle of the animal. Make use of whatever is available as a weapon.

To protect both you and the bear, you must react calmly and intelligently if you come across one in the wild. You can adapt your activities to the bear's behavior by determining if it is curious, defensive, or predatory. Remain composed, identify yourself, and, when it's safe to do so, take a cautious step back.

In bear encounters, bear spray is an essential tool since it offers a non-lethal way to dissuade hostile bears. Accurate aim, controlled bursts, and knowledge of the bear spray's effective range are all necessary for its proper application.

Bear spray should be used soon after the occurrence, and local authorities should be notified.

Anybody going into bear country needs to be able to read bear body language. By observing posture, movement, vocalizations, and eye contact, you may identify signals of curiosity, defensiveness, and predation. This will help you respond effectively and lower the possibility of an escalation.

The essentials to safe outdoor excursions are preparedness, education, and respect. You may reduce the chance of bear encounters and responsibly and securely enjoy nature by being aware of bear habits, carrying and using bear spray, and interpreting body language.

Surviving A Bear Attack

Bear attacks are uncommon, but they can happen, and being prepared might be the difference between life and death. This chapter examines the many bear attack scenarios, including defensive and predatory attacks, and offers comprehensive advice on surviving a run-in with a black, grizzly, or polar bear.

It also discusses playing dead and when and how to use it as a tactic to improve your chances of surviving.

Predatory vs. Defensive Attacks

Determining the proper response to a bear assault requires an understanding of its motives.

1. Defensive Strikes

Cause: A bear will launch a defensive attack if it perceives a threat or is cornered. This might occur if you unexpectedly come across a bear, get too close to one, or unintentionally get in the way of a mother grizzly and her kids.

Behavior: Before making physical contact, defensive bears may use warning signs like puffing, clacking their teeth, or bluff charging to try to scare you away.

Response: Talk in a soothing, calm voice, be composed, don't move suddenly, and back away gradually. Avoid looking someone in the eye or acting hostilely.

2. Attacks by Predators

Cause: When a bear perceives you as food, it will attack you predatorily. A bear may do this if it is ill, food-conditioned, or experiencing extreme hunger as a result of its surroundings.

Behavior: Predatory bears may stalk in a stealthy, steady manner, moving with determination and attention. They are not as likely to display warning symptoms before striking.

Reaction: Be confident, project as much size and might as you can, and get ready to launch a forceful self-defense. To survive a predatory attack, you might need to fight back.

How to Respond to an Attack by a Black Bear

Even though black bears are often less hostile than grizzly bears, they can still be dangerous, particularly if they sense danger or have become accustomed to food.

1. Remain composed.

Try not to panic if a black bear charges or approaches you. Stay composed.

2. Make a Huge Difference for Yourself

To project an imposing and larger-than-life image of yourself, stand tall and wave your arms above your head.

3. Return Gradually

Face the beast and slowly retreat. Avoid turning around or running since this may result in a pursuit reaction.

4. Apply bear repellent

Use bear spray as a deterrent if the bear keeps coming. For best results, aim for the bear's eyes and face.

5. Retaliate if Needed

If the bear attacks, retaliate forcefully with whatever weapons or items you have on hand. The bear's face and muzzle are the most susceptible spots to attack.

How to Respond to an Attack by a Grizzly Bear

Because grizzly bears are bigger and more ferocious than black bears, interactions with them may be riskier.

1. Evaluate the circumstances

Ascertain whether the bear is behaving aggressively or defensively. A lowered head, relaxed ears, and aggressive vocalizations are examples of aggressive signals.

2. Act Dead or Resist

Play dead by lying face down with your hands clasped behind your neck if the bear is displaying defensive behavior. To make it more difficult for the bear to turn you over, spread your legs. Until the bear departs the area, remain motionless.

Use any accessible weapons or objects to respond forcefully if the bear is behaving aggressively and shows no indications of stopping. Target the face and muzzle of the bear.

3. Apply bear repellent

Use bear spray as a deterrent if you have any. For best results, aim for the bear's eyes and face.

How to Handle an Attack by a Polar Bear

Because of the bears' size and predatory instincts, encounters with polar bears are uncommon but can be very deadly.

1. Evaluate the circumstances

Ascertain whether the bear is behaving aggressively or defensively. Because polar bears are inherently hunters, they may perceive humans as prey.

2. Apply bear repellent

Use bear spray as a deterrent if you have any. For best results, aim for the bear's eyes and face.

3. Strike Back Hard

If the bear attacks, retaliate forcefully with whatever weapons or items you have on hand. The bear's face and muzzle are the most susceptible spots to attack.

4. If at all possible, seek refuge

Try to go to a car or shelter as soon as you can if you're near one. Despite their considerable swimming ability, polar bears can be discouraged by small areas or obstructions.

Playing Dead: When and How

The last resort in a defensive grizzly bear attack situation is to play dead. Here's when and how to use this strategy:

1. When to Act Mortal

Only pretend to be dead if you are positive the bear is defending itself and isn't attempting to pounce on you. A lack of predatory behavior, protective vocalizations, and bluff charges are some telltale signals to watch out for.

2. Take Up the Role

To safeguard your important organs, lay face down with your hands clasped behind your neck. To make it more difficult for the bear to turn you over, spread your legs.

3. Remain motionless and quiet.

Try to be as still and quiet as you can. Avoid making any abrupt movements or noises that can agitate the bear even more.

4. Hold off until the bear departs.

Continue acting as though you're dead until the bear moves on. Stay alert and don't move until you are positive the bear has left.

Extra Techniques to Withstand a Bear Attack

Apart from the particular techniques delineated for distinct kinds of bear encounters, there exist other overarching strategies that can augment your odds of enduring a bear assault.

Get Ready

Always Carry Bear Deterrents: When traveling through bear country, be sure you have bear spray or other deterrents on hand. Ensure that it's simple to use and become knowledgeable about its capabilities.

Travel in Groups: It is less common for bears to approach human groups. Along with increasing safety, traveling in groups can help avoid encounters with bears.

Make Noise: If a bear hears people approaching, it will usually steer clear. When trekking, make noise, particularly in places with a lot of forest or poor sight.

Remain Alert: Pay attention to your surroundings and keep an eye out for any indications of bear activity, such as footprints, scat, or overturned boulders.

Recognize Your Environment

Prevent Unexpected Meetings: Exercise extra caution while traversing regions with poor visibility, such as dense underbrush or trail bends. To let bears know you're around, make noise.

Remain Away from Bear Food Sources: Steer clear of locations where there are clear indications of bear activity, like feeding grounds or carcasses. In areas where berries, streams for fishing, or other natural food sources are present, exercise extra caution.

Select Safe Campsites: Stay away from paths and water sources while selecting a campsite in the bar area. Stay away from preparing and keeping food close to where you sleep.

React Suitably

Remain Calm: Try not to flinch or become agitated if you come upon a bear. Bears are fearful and may defend themselves.

Evaluate the Situation: Quickly ascertain whether the bear is acting in a protective or predatory manner based on its behavior. Your answer will be determined by this.

When retreating from a bear that is on the defense, take your time and face the animal. Refrain from running or turning around as this could lead to an attack.

Use Bear Spray: If the bear keeps coming near or exhibits aggressive behavior, use bear spray. For best results, aim for the bear's eyes and face.

Fight Back: Retaliate violently and with all the tools at your disposal if a bear attacks. Since the bear's face and muzzle are its most susceptible spots, target them.

Get Medical Help

Seek Medical Assistance: Even if your wounds appear to be minor, you should get medical assistance as soon as possible after surviving a bear assault. Serious injuries from bear attacks can include lacerations and puncture wounds, which call for immediate medical attention.

Report the Incident: Notify the park rangers or the local wildlife authority about the bear attack. This may stop more attacks and aid in tracking bear behavior.

Take Away Knowledge from the Experience

Consider the Encounter: Give the bear encounter some thought and consider the lessons you can draw from it. Think about what worked and what you could have done differently to enhance your response in similar situations in the future.

Educate Others: Talk about your bear encounters with others to spread the word about bear safety and the value of being ready when visiting bear territory. Motivate people to educate themselves about bear behavior and appropriate responses when facing bears.

It takes a combination of alertness, readiness, and fast thinking to survive a bear assault. By implementing these extra precautions and maintaining composure in stressful situations, you can improve your odds of surviving a bear encounter with little damage.

Bears are wild animals, so interactions with them can be erratic. Keep that in mind. When you are in bear country, respect their space, be ready for anything, and put safety first.

You can enjoy the environment and reduce the chance of encountering bears while also making sure that everyone has a safe and enjoyable outdoor experience if you have the appropriate information and mindset.

Tools And Safety Equipment

Having the proper tools and safety gear can make all the difference in assuring a fun and safe outdoor experience when heading into bear country. This covers basic safety equipment such as bear spray, noise-producing gadgets, fences and containers that are bear-proof, and personal protection tools like guns and substitutes.

Devices for Creating Noise: Air Horns, Whistles, and Bells

1. Rings of Bears

Bear bells are made to make noise while you travel, which is intended to alert bears to your presence. Providing bears with an opportunity to detect your approach is intended to avert unexpected meetings.

Effectiveness: Bear bells have some effect in open areas, but their usefulness may be diminished in thick vegetation due to sound bafflement. In these circumstances, it is still imperative to maintain vigilance and generate more noise.

2. Horns

The purpose of whistles is to serve as a signaling device in an emergency by being lightweight and compact, which makes them convenient to carry. Bears can be made aware of your presence by using them as well.

High-Pitched noises: Whistles and other high-pitched noises may be more successful at warning bears than other noise-making objects because bears may be more sensitive to these sounds.

3. Air Horns

The goal of air horns is to scare and discourage bears with their piercing, loud sound. Compared to bear bells or whistles, they have a greater range of effectiveness.

One-Time Use: Since air horns are usually only meant to be used once, they might not be the best option for lengthy excursions into bear territory. They may be helpful, nevertheless, in an emergency or as temporary deterrents.

Bear-Proof Fences and Containers

1. Bear-Resistant Containers

The goal of bear-proof containers is to keep food, garbage, and other smelly objects safely stored away from bears. To reduce confrontations between humans and bears and prevent bears from connecting humans with food, proper food storage is essential.

Types: Bear-resistant canisters, locked coolers, and hanging food bags are a few examples of bear-proof container designs. Select a container that satisfies the particular needs of your journey and destination.

2. Electric Fencing

The goal of electric fences is to erect a barrier that keeps bears out of specific areas, like campgrounds and food storage facilities. They deter bears from trying to scale the fence by shocking them with a moderate electric jolt when they come into contact.

Options for Portability: Temporary use of electric fences in rural environments is possible with portable models. In Bear Country, they offer additional safety for campers and backpackers and are lightweight and simple to set up.

3. How to Use Bear-Proof Fences and Containers Properly

Food and fragrant products should always be stored in bear-proof containers or hung from a bear-resistant food-hanging system to ensure food safety. Never leave these things unattended in your car or when camping.

Respect Instructions: When utilizing electric fences, pay attention to the installation and maintenance instructions provided by the manufacturer. Make sure the fence is installed properly, and test it frequently to make sure it's operating as intended.

Handguns and Other Options for Personal Protection

1. Weapons

Goal: For personal defense against bear attacks, some people view firearms as a last-resort measure. When utilized properly, they can be useful in halting a bear that is charging.

Considerations: It takes practice, training, and knowledge of local rules and ordinances to use a firearm for bear defense. Forbear protection, select a suitable caliber and load, and be ready to employ it with effectiveness in a high-stress scenario.

2. Things to Think About with Firearms

Know How to Use It: Getting the right instruction in the handling and upkeep of a handgun is crucial if you decide to carry one for bear protection. Learn the rules and restrictions in your area about carrying and using a firearm when you're in bear country.

Carry Caution: It's important to use caution when carrying a gun. Make sure you're emotionally and psychologically ready to utilize it in a life-threatening emergency. To stay proficient, practice drawing and aiming your pistol frequently.

Bear Spray: When it comes to preventing bear attacks, bear spray is usually thought to be more useful and effective than guns.

It is simple to employ, non-lethal, and has a track record of successfully discouraging hostile bears.

Whistles, air horns, and other noise-making tools can be useful deterrents for frightening off bears in non-life-threatening circumstances. Bears may be startled and deterred from coming any closer by them.

To reduce the chances of bear encounters and guarantee a safe outdoor experience in bear territory, safety gear and gadgets are essential. The most popular deterrent against bear assaults is bear spray, which should be carried and used according to manufacturer instructions.

Guns are one type of personal protection that should be used sensibly and with considerable thought. Whenever feasible, bear deterrence should give preference to non-lethal techniques to encourage harmonious cohabitation between people and bears in their natural habitat.

3. Use Bear Spray Carefully

Accessibility: Always have your bear spray close at hand, ideally in a holster fastened to the strap of your backpack or belt. Should an encounter arise, you should be able to draw it fast.

Practice Deployment: Become acquainted with how to use your bear spray. To be sure you can launch the canister in a high-stress scenario, practice removing the safety clip and aiming it.

Verify the Expiration Dates: The shelf life of bear spray is normally three to four years. To guarantee its efficacy, frequently check the expiration date and replace the canister as needed.

4. Utilizing Noise-Making Devices Efficiently

Change Up Your Sounds: Bear bells are a great way to let bears know you're there, but you should also change up your sounds to keep them from getting too repetitive. Bear bells can be combined with sporadic cries or whistles to produce a variety of sounds.

Remain Aware: Noise-generating devices, such as bear bells, are not infallible. Stay alert and keep an eye out for indications of bear activity, particularly in places with a lot of foliage or poor visibility.

To reduce the likelihood of bear encounters and guarantee a secure outdoor experience in bear territory, safety gear and gadgets are indispensable. The most effective method of deterring bears is still bear spray, which should be carried and used responsibly according to manufacturer instructions.

Bears can be scared off by using noise-making tools like air horns, bear bells, and whistles to let them know you are there. Nonetheless, they must be kept up with situational awareness and utilized in concert with additional safety precautions.

To lessen the possibility of human-bear confrontations, bears cannot access food or scented goods, hence bear-proof containers and electric fences are essential.

Guns and other personal defense equipment should be used sensibly and with caution; if feasible, non-lethal solutions should be prioritized.

You may enjoy the woods responsibly and safely, even in bear country, if you have the proper safety gear, tools, and knowledge about bear behavior and safety precautions.

First Aid for Bear Encounters

Injuries from encounters with bears in the wild can range from small scratches and bruises to more serious wounds. It's critical to know how to provide basic first aid for injuries sustained in a bear attack to protect both yourself and other people.

Additionally, minimizing additional harm following a bear encounter can be achieved by being aware of the concepts of emergency reaction and evacuation. The psychological fallout from bear encounters is also covered in this chapter, along with advice on how to cope with trauma and get help.

Basic Medical Care for Bear Attack Victims

1. Evaluate the circumstances

Assure Safety: Make sure the location is free of any imminent risks, such as other bears or environmental hazards, before providing first aid.

Examine Injuries: Determine the type and extent of wounds received during the bear encounter. Sort treatments according to the victim's state and the extent of their wounds.

2. Put an end to the bleeding

Apply Pressure: Apply direct pressure to any bleeding wounds using a clean cloth or bandages. If at all feasible, elevate the wounded limb to assist in reducing blood flow.

Use a tourniquet: To stop the blood supply to the injured limb in cases of serious bleeding that cannot be stopped with pressure, think about applying a tourniquet. Make sure the tourniquet is tight enough to halt the bleeding without inflicting more damage before applying it above the wound.

3. Clean and Tidy Injuries

Cleanse Wounds: To lower the chance of infection, give any wounds a thorough cleaning with soap and water. If available, use a saline solution to irrigate the wounds.

Apply Dressings: To prevent infection, cover the wounds with sterile dressings or a clean piece of cloth. Bandages or sticky tape can be used to keep the dressings in place.

4. Handle with Shock

Maintain Warmth: Provide warmth and comfort to the person if they exhibit symptoms of shock, such as pale skin, a fast heartbeat, or shallow breathing. To keep their bodies warm, cover them with jackets or blankets.

Legs Up: Raise the victim's legs a little to enhance blood supply to essential organs and lower the chance of fainting.

Evacuation and Emergency Response

1. Make a Help Request

Contact Emergency Services: To request medical attention and an evacuation, try to contact emergency services by phone or by asking for help from people in the vicinity.

Give accurate Location Information: To help rescuers find you, give them accurate location information such as GPS coordinates, trails, or landmarks.

2. Go to safety and evacuate

Transfer to a Safe Area: If the bear encounter happened in a distant wilderness area, you might want to relocate to a more secure spot that isn't near the bear's home range.

Assist injured parties: Assist wounded parties in moving to a safe location, being cautious to support any sprained limbs and prevent exacerbating their injuries.

3. Keep an eye out for complications

Watch for Infection Symptoms: Keep an eye out for symptoms of infection in injured people, such as elevated pain, swelling, redness, or discharge coming from wounds. Seek quick medical assistance if infection symptoms appear.

Keep an Eye Out for Psychological suffering: Observe both the injured persons and other group members for indications of psychological suffering, such as worry, fear, or symptoms of post-traumatic stress disorder.

Psychological Repercussions: Handling Trauma

1. Offer Support on an Emotional Level

Offer Reassurance: Assure those impacted by the bear encounter and extend emotional assistance. Acknowledge their emotions and lend a sympathetic ear.

Promote Open Communication: Promote honest dialogue regarding the encounter, giving people a safe space to share their feelings, ideas, and worries.

2. Seek Expert Assistance

Counseling Services: If you or a loved one is suffering from severe psychological discomfort or trauma associated with the bear experience, you might think about getting professional counseling or therapy.

Support Groups: Make contact with online forums or support groups for others who have gone through comparable traumatic experiences. Talking to people about your experiences and coping mechanisms can be a great way to get support and validation.

3. Take Care of Yourself

Practice Relaxation Techniques: To help people cope with stress and anxiety, encourage them to use relaxation techniques like progressive muscle relaxation, deep breathing, and meditation.

Maintain Routine: To foster a sense of normalcy and well-being, encourage people to carry out their favorite activities and stick to their regular schedules.

4. Examine for injuries to the head and neck

Examine for Head Injuries: If the victim's head was struck during the bear encounter, pay close attention to any indications of a head injury, such as dizziness, nausea, or loss of consciousness. Keep a watchful eye on the victim in case their consciousness or behavior changes.

Maintain Neck Stabilization: Refrain from moving the victim's head or neck if there is a possibility of a neck injury. Using the proper support, such as rolled towels or garments on either side of the head, stabilize the neck.

5. Offer consolation and assurance

Remain Calm: To comfort the injured person and anyone nearby, maintain your composure. Your manner can foster a sense of security and lessen tension.

Provide Emotional Support: Pay close attention to the hurt person's worries and offer consoling and uplifting remarks. Reassure them that they are not alone and that assistance is on its way.

Observe Directions: Pay attention to the guidance given by first responders or emergency dispatchers. They might provide instructions on how to stabilize the wounded party and get ready to leave.

Inform Emergency Services of Any Changes: Report to them any modifications to the victim's condition or the surrounding area. Responders can use this information to evaluate the situation and offer the right kind of aid.

6. Put the evacuation plan into action.

Transport Efficiently: If evacuation is required, collaborate with other group members to transport the injured person safely and effectively. If there are any available, transfer the sufferer using stretchers or makeshift carriers.

Remain Vigilant: Throughout the evacuation procedure, remain mindful of any potential dangers, such as uneven ground, impediments, or bad weather. Take safety measures to protect the injured person and the rescuers.

7. Encourage Resilience

Encourage people to concentrate on the coping mechanisms and assets that have previously enabled them to overcome obstacles. Remind them of their tenacity and capacity to handle challenging circumstances.